GET MOVING AGAIN

Constipation is one of those problems no one wants to talk about, yet all of us suffer from it, if only just occasionally. Many people cannot achieve normal elimination without the regular use of laxatives, which in itself can lead to other serious health problems. Studies show that 70 to 80 percent of colon cancer is caused by diet and poor bowel habits. Approximately 100 million Americans suffer from some sort of digestive disturbance, resulting in an estimated loss in wages and medical costs of over $50 billion. Quite simply, good colon health is essential to overall good health. By suggesting simple changes in diet and lifestyle, this helpful booklet empowers the reader to solve this uncomfortable problem once and for all.

ABOUT THE AUTHOR

Donna DiMarco is a licensed nutrition counselor with a practice in South Florida. She hosts a local weekly radio talk show on health and nutrition. Besides regularly lecturing on nutrition topics, Donna writes a weekly health column, has formulated several nutritional products, and serves on the board of directors of the Florida Nutrition Counselors Association.

ACKNOWLEDGMENTS

I am so thankful for all the help, encouragement, and support from my daughters Stacy and Dana, my friends Meir and Angela Pear, Tom Dynan, and Dorothy Leibowitz, and my favorite artist, Tom Cavanagh, who has shown me that he (and I) can do all things and overcome all obstacles if we set our minds to it and trust God. Thanks to you all!

Natural Relief from Constipation

Using Herbal Remedies, Diet, and Exercise to Promote Good Colon Health and Restore Balance to the Body

by Donna DiMarco

KEATS PUBLISHING

LOS ANGELES

NTC/Contemporary Publishing Group

DEDICATION

To my sister, Betty Kennedy, who avoided colorectal surgery by taking my advice just days before the scheduled hospitalization. I'm glad I could help, Bebe!

Natural Relief from Constipation is intended solely for informational and educational purposes and not as medical advice. Please consult a medical or health professional if you have questions about your health.

NATURAL RELIEF FROM CONSTIPATION

Published by Keats
A division of NTC/Contemporary Publishing Group, Inc.
4255 West Touhy Avenue, Lincolnwood (Chicago), Illinois 60712, U.S.A.
Copyright © 1999 by Donna DiMarco
Printed and bound in the United States of America
International Standard Book Number: 0-87983-958-9

7 8 9 0 DIG /DIG 16 15 14 13

Contents

Millions of people suffer from constipation. It is no laughing matter, though jokes and smirks occur whenever this embarrassing topic is mentioned. But it must be addressed, because without regular and comfortable bowel habits, good health cannot be achieved.

It is believed that 80 to 90 percent of Americans suffer from constipation and its debilitating effects, which cause one to feel heavy and sluggish, weighed down, and in slow motion both physically and mentally. Moreover, constipation often leads to other health problems such as headaches, diverticulosis, PMS, bad breath, canker sores, body odor, hemorrhoids, varicose veins, malabsorption, obesity, indigestion, and the most deadly outcome, colon cancer.

Fecal waste is a normal by-product of digestion, but it must be eliminated because it is toxic and can breed pathogens such as yeast and bacteria, which themselves can cause further problems. Research has shown that these antigens and toxins may play a role in the development of what appear to be totally unrelated diseases such as diabetes mellitus, migraine headaches, myasthenia gravis, meningitis, and thyroid disease. Nearly twenty years ago, the prestigious medical journal, the *Lancet*, reported that women who have two or fewer bowel movements per week have four times the risk of breast disease (benign or malignant) as women who have one or more bowel movements per day.

Constipation is the buildup of digestive by-products in the colon. If fecal waste moves too slowly out of the body, elimination becomes difficult, causing increased pressure in the abdomen. The belly can feel hard and distended by the extra mass that is retained. An increase of gas can occur, creating further distension and more pressure within the colon. This increase in intraintestinal pressure can cause the outpouching of the colon wall (diverticulae); fecal matter can eventually get stuck in these pouches, which become inflamed. This is known as *diverticulitis*. The increased abdominal pressure can also bring about a slowdown in the movement of food through the digestive tract, which results in a backup in the entire digestive canal. If this backup occurs frequently, hernias can occur at the various sphincters located throughout the digestive canal. If the urge to evacuate is great, but the stool is too hard, dry, or large, the pressure on the rectum and anus can lead to hemorrhoids or piles. If one tries to eliminate these hard, dry stools, tiny tears may occur in the delicate tissue of the rectum.

There are thus a lot of good reasons to keep things moving out of the body. Just as in life—the longer we hold on to the digestive or other by-products of the past, the less we can enjoy the things of the present. Think about it!

CAUSES

Constipation can have a variety of causes:

- Diseases of the anus and rectum, such as diverticulitis, tumors, or rectoceles (outpouching of the rectal wall)

- Spinal cord injury
- Neurological disorders such as Hirschsprung's disease
- Low levels of thyroid hormone
- High levels of calcium
- Medications such as calcium channel blockers, antidepressants, antacids, antihistamines, morphine, colchicine, some arthritis medications, anticholinergics for treatment of schizophrenia, and antiemetics.
- Diabetes and kidney failure
- Pregnancy (due to the pressure of the baby on the mother's rectum)
- Psychological difficulties that arise in childhood from inappropriate toilet training
- Stress and tension
- Change of environment when traveling
- Regularly ignoring to the body's signals to defecate
- Too little water, too little dietary fiber, not enough exercise
- Food sensitivities (see page 32)

THE INTESTINAL TRACT

The intestinal tract is a hollow tube beginning at the mouth and ending at the anus; a lot of important activity occurs in between. The function of the digestive tract is to convert food into a form that can be used more readily by the body. Digestion begins in the mouth, where chewing breaks the food down into small pieces. With the help of the tongue, the food mixes with saliva into a semiliquid to pass down the gullet. This semiliquid, or *chyme*, allows the food to mix more thoroughly with the digestive enzymes needed to further digest it. The saliva contains the enzymes salivary amylase and lingual lipase, which quickly begin the breakdown of carbohydrates and fat. The chyme is now ready to pass through the esophagus and into the stomach.

The stomach is a pouch-shaped organ with a strong mucous lining, which protects it from digesting itself. The surface area of the stomach is increased by the presence of folds within its cavity called *ruggae*. The ruminating within the folds helps to mix the food with stomach secretions. The stomach produces hydrochloric acid from the parietal cells within its walls, which help denature protein; that is, the acid in the stomach helps to gently unwrap the coils of the protein bonds so that the other protein-digesting enzymes can break it down into its smallest, most usable form. Stomach acid is important for good health, as it helps mineral absorption and kills the bacteria and parasites that may accompany the food.

Occasionally, one may feel burning in the stomach and conclude that the body is producing too much acid. Very often, the opposite is true. The lack of hydrochloric acid can produce a burning feeling similar to that produced by too much acid. The acid environment of the stomach is necessary to trigger the production of alkaline substances in the next stage of digestion, in the small intestine. The consistent use of antacids actually hinders the digestive process. Without acid breakdown, the food is not in an absorbable form, and this may very well set the stage for future health problems. When there is a large amount of fat or fiber in a meal, food will stay in the stomach longer than if it is composed of mostly simple carbohydrates. Generally speaking, food remains in the stomach for two to four hours.

The same parietal cells that produce hydrochloric acid also produce *intrinsic factor*, which helps us absorb vitamin B_{12} further down the intestinal tract. If we are producing too little hydrochloric acid, chances are we are producing too little intrinsic factor, which may lead to pernicious anemia. As we get older, we automatically produce less hydrochloric acid and intrinsic factor. This explains why so many older people do well with B_{12} shots for that little bit of extra energy and enhanced mental acuity.

The stomach also produces *pepsin* to aid in protein digestion and small amounts of a fat-digesting enzyme called *lipase*, but generally, most protein and fat digestion occurs in the small intestine. (The only thing absorbed in the stomach is ethyl alcohol, the type found in alcoholic beverages. This accounts for the rapid increase in blood alcohol levels soon after a drink or two is consumed. Drinking alcoholic beverages after eating will slow down the alcohol absorption rate.) When sufficient mixing of food and enzymes has occurred, the partially digested food passes from the stomach, through the *pyloric valve*, and into the *duodenum*.

The duodenum is the first eight to sixteen inches of the small intestine, which wraps around the head of the pancreas to connect to the jejunum. The duodenum produces both *secretin*, which stimulates the duodenal juices, and *cholecystokinin* that causes the gall bladder to contract, providing bile salts and enzymes to further aid in digestion. The duodenum has a tiny sensor to detect the pH (acidity and alkalinity) of the chyme. If it is sufficiently acidic, the duodenum tells the body to send out, in essence, "baking soda" to neutralize the acid so further digestion can occur in a more alkaline environment. If the chyme is not acidic enough, then less "baking soda" is released and the chyme remains acidic. Food in this form cannot be broken down into its smaller parts for absorption. The digestive process slows down, and nutrients that would have passed into the body after digestion remain in a partially digested state in the intestinal tract.

If this partially digested food stays in the intestines too long, it tends to putrefy or rot. Imagine a can that is bulging at the lid due to internal pressure from spoiled food. Just as in the can, gas is produced, and a very unfavorable environment occurs. We've all experienced intestinal gas. If it occurs in the upper digestive tract, it can escape as a belch or a burp; in the lower intestines, it makes its presence known as flatulence. Actually, a small amount of gas is normal, but excessive amounts can cause cramping and abdominal discomfort. By insuring a proper pH in the stomach, we can encourage efficient digestion in the small intestine. The duodenum is the location of pancreatic enzyme secretions for the digestion of fats, proteins, and carbohydrates.

The liver plays a part in this process, too. It is in this area that the common bile duct joins with the pancreatic duct at the Ampulla of Vater. Bile produced in the liver flows into the duodenum to help break down fat and cholesterol. It also helps protect the small intestine from the strong stomach acid by providing substantial amounts of buffering bicarbonates.

In the next eight to ten feet of the small intestine, called the *jejunum,* some sugars, some water-soluble B vitamins, and proteins and amino acids are absorbed. Chyme stays in the small intestine for approximately three to six hours before passing into the ileum.

Most absorption of nutrients occurs in the duodenum and jejunum. The duodenum is responsible for the absorption of fats, minerals, some simple sugars, some B vitamins, and vitamin C, as well as the fat-soluble vitamins A, D, E, and K.

The distal three-fifths of the small intestine is called the *ileum,* where bile salts, vitamin B_{12}, and cholesterol are absorbed. The length of the ileum can vary from fifteen to thirty feet, depending on the person's size. In the lower right corner of the abdomen, the ileum joins the large intestines at the *ileocecal valve.*

The large intestine is between three to five feet in length and encircles the abdominal perimeter. It meets with an S-shaped tube called the *sigmoid* and ends with the *rectum,* then the *anus.* Constipation sometimes occurs due to the severe curves of the sigmoid. Years ago, our ancestors overcame this by squatting in the woods using muscles in the sigmoid as well as the rectum to defecate. Our modern-day toilets are designed for us to sit down, keeping us from using our anatomy properly and possibly causing bowel problems.

The colon is where water absorption takes place. Electrolytes such as sodium and potassium are absorbed here as well, but that isn't its only function. Good bacteria (probiotics) in the colon are essential for health, and these friendly critters help maintain a favorable environment by keeping bad bacteria and yeast in check. They also help with absorption of nutrients, conversion of vitamins K and B from their precursors, stimulation of the immune system, provision of proper motility in the colon, and production of short-chained fatty acids, especially butyric acid, all of which are necessary for colon health.

Problems can occur at any point in the digestive tract, provoking symptoms that may be obvious or may appear to be totally unrelated. For example, insufficient stomach acid can be linked to eczema, food allergies, or osteoporosis. The proper tests can easily identify the underlying causes of these and most other health problems. A wonderful Web site that is geared to the layperson but specific enough for the practitioner is operated by Great Smokies Diagnostic Laboratory (www.greatsmokies-lab.com); it can direct the reader to the proper diagnostic tools to identify most problems. Great Smokies does a variety of testing but is particularly impressive at diagnosing gastrointestinal disorders. The Comprehensive Digestive Stool Analysis (CDSA) is a simple stool sampling that is more comprehensive than what your doctor may routinely order. A practitioner must order the CDSA, but this Web site will give you all the information to bring to your practitioner. I strongly encourage you to check it out.

WHAT IS NORMAL?

FREQUENCY

The frequency of bowel movements varies from person to person. Some people go two to three times each day, and others consider once or twice a week standard. Most medical professionals feel that whatever is normal for you is what you should expect. Holistic doctors and nutritionists don't agree. Because we consume food several times each day, the transit time (the time from when you eat until the food's waste materials pass out of the body) should be less than twenty-four hours to keep toxins from building up and distending the colon. A longer time can cause a backup, creating toxic by-products while giving anaerobic bacteria a chance to flourish. If we keep packing food into the intestines without letting any (or very little) out, the colon will stretch to accommodate the increased volume. Fecal matter is packed against the intestinal walls, rendering the microscopic fingerlike projections (villi) that increase surface absorption useless. This coating on the intestinal tract hinders peristalsis (the wavelike contractions of the intestinal muscles that help keep wastes moving and eventually evacuated), which in itself slows down bowel transit time. The longer the waste stays in the colon, the more water is absorbed from it, so the harder it becomes. The harder it becomes, the more difficult it is to eliminate, creating a vicious cycle. Intestinal transit time can be easily tracked by consuming beets or corn on the cob; note the time and day the food is eaten and notice when you see the residual passed out of the body in the stool.

There is more to normal bowel movements than just frequency. There are other factors to consider: What color is the stool? What is its consistency? Does it sink or float? Is there a lot of bowel gas? Is there a foul odor? Is there any visible blood or mucus?

COLOR

Color is important because it can indicate good bowel health or possible problems. A normal stool should be a walnut brown. A light stool might indicate a liver problem. A black stool might mean there may be bleeding higher up in the digestive tract, very often caused by a bleeding ulcer or other serious problem. It might also indicate, however, that you are taking an iron supplement, or chlorella, or have had a green drink. If you are not consuming any of these, call your physician for an appointment as soon as possible. Eating beets might turn your stool red the next day or so, but a bright red blood color is a signal to call your physician immediately.

CONSISTENCY

The consistency of a healthy bowel movement should be similar to toothpaste, formed and lengthy, not little hard pellets like rabbits produce. Sometimes these pellets form a larger mass that becomes difficult to expel. That's just the built-up pieces of stool being pressed into each other. This may indicate that you're not digesting as well as you should. Each section of stool should be, for the most part, homogeneous and long. It should be about the length and shape of a good-sized banana, though not necessarily as wide. You may pass several sections like this, depending on the amount of fiber in your diet and the how much food you've eaten.

SINK OR SWIM?

Does your stool sink or float? If there is not enough fiber in your diet, your stool will quickly plummet to the bottom of the bowl. On the other hand, if every bit of excrement floats on top of the water, you might have too much fiber in your diet, although this is rarely the case. Floating stools may also be an indication of pancreatic disease. Normal stool will settle into the water and the increased volume may cause it to sink, but not totally out of sight. It should be large enough to represent the amount of food eaten, yet pass easily out of the body with little effort, and it should be well formed. Although the mass of waste might cause some to remain above the water level, it should basically be submerged.

Dietary adjustments are easy to make to increase your fiber intake—simply eat more fresh fruits and vegetables. Plant foods are better than fiber supplements, since they provide not only fiber but also phytonutrients to prevent disease and maintain health. If the body doesn't respond to an increase in dietary fiber, then consider adding fiber in a supplemental form: pill, capsule, wafer, or powder. Sometimes psyllium husks or other supplemental fibers bring with them the embarrassing problem of flatulence. If large amounts of fiber are taken all at once, the body reacts by producing extra gas. This is common and can be overcome simply by starting with a small amount of fiber (about one-half teaspoon) and gradually increasing it as the digestive system adjusts. It is essential to drink adequate amounts of water when taking fiber supplements.

BOWEL GAS

Bowel gas is a normal occurrence. Sometimes we swallow air when we eat, especially if we eat too fast. Sometimes gas comes in with our foods, as with carbonated beverages. Certain foods such as beans, peppers, and brewer's yeast can stimulate the production of bowel gas.

If you have an explosion every time you have a bowel movement, however, or malodorous gas sneaks out of you at the most inappropriate times, you may need to make some changes in diet, supplements, lifestyle, or a combination of these. If digestion is impaired, whether it is from diet, improper food combining, stress, medication, or over-the-counter remedies, the food ferments, giving off gas. Carbon dioxide, which is harmless, makes up a lot of it. Ammonia is also produced and is mostly absorbed into the blood to be excreted in the urine, but some passes out as flatus. Hydrogen sulfide and methane are exclusively passed via the anus. You can blame the hydrogen sulfide for the unpleasant odor that's a sure giveaway of your digestive insufficiencies. A healthy bowel movement has a slight but not overpowering smell; if it's unpleasantly strong, it's an indication that your diet and digestive system are out of balance. Very often the culprit is combining protein and carbohydrates in the same meal, leading to improper digestion and flatulence.

Everyone suffers from flatulence from time to time. Some of us have smelly bowel movements once in a while, and lots of people have stools that sink invisibly to the bottom of the bowl; that's okay if it is occasional and not your normal function. The goal of this booklet is to teach you how to read these indicators of what's happening within your body, then take the appropriate actions to correct the situation and restore health.

WHAT IS WRONG WITH LAXATIVES?

The word *laxative* comes from the Latin word *laxare*, which means to loosen. *Taber's Cyclopedic Medical Dictionary* defines it as "a mild purgative medicine; an aperient or mild cathartic." These so-called mild medicines, however, often prompt us to madly dash to the nearest rest room. The opposite is also true. Sometimes, laxatives don't do a thing, and you are left feeling bloated and uncomfortable.

If we repeatedly rely on laxatives to have bowel movements, the tiny muscles surrounding the bowel become weak from disuse. Eventually, they atrophy and actually cannot function. After long-term use of laxatives, peristaltic contractions become weak, and the colon loses its ability to constrict and relax to move the fecal matter out of the body. If you have become dependent on laxatives, a high-fiber diet, copious water consumption, and regular exercise can encourage restoration of normal function.

Too often, people who suffer from constipation take a laxative for quick relief. This may be helpful at the time, but since the cause of the constipation was not addressed, constipation may occur again. If it does, another laxative is usually taken to remedy the problem. This scenario may be repeated over and over until the only way a person can have a bowel movement is by taking laxatives on a regular basis. Eventually, a single dose of laxative becomes ineffective so more than the recommended dose is taken. Soon this larger dose becomes necessary just to maintain regular bowel movements. At this point, a laxative habit, or an addiction of sorts, has developed and can be very difficult to break.

Some young women are so concerned with their appearance that they use laxatives as a weight-reduction method, believing that they can consume whatever they like and then take large doses of laxatives so that the calories aren't absorbed. The problem is that nutrients aren't absorbed either. Studies indicate that laxative abuse can lead to hypokalemia (potassium deficiency) caused by the loss of body fluids through frequent evacuation. This can cause damage of the renal tubules and possibly even kidney failure due to profound fluid volume depletion. This loss of gastrointestinal fluid reduces the volume of urine, leaving uric acid and ammonium acid urate to form stones in the genitourinary tract. Anyone who has ever experienced a kidney stone will attest to the severity of the pain.

With long-term laxative use, the body's pH becomes quite alkaline, which can affect many body functions. Habitual laxative abuse can lead to morphological changes in the autonomic nervous system of the colon. It has also been noted that the macrophages within the submucosa of the colon can become dark in color as a result of laxative abuse. A Swiss study determined that long-term abuse of laxatives could lead to irritable colon, which manifests as chronic diarrhea and is very difficult to treat. In addition, an article by C. P. Sieger and colleagues in the British journal *Gut* concluded in 1993 that anthranoid-containing laxatives, such as cascara sagrada, aloe vera, and frangula, might be implicated in colorectal cancer. That's a high price to pay for relying on laxatives.

Laxatives, even natural ones, can cause inflammation of the intestinal wall, deplete much-needed electrolytes, and permanently damage the delicate mucosal lining of the intestinal tract. Long-term use may even lead to mucosal necrosis (deadening of the intestinal lining), kidney damage, or possibly cancer. Occasional laxative use may sometimes be necessary, but don't let it become a habit. Learn to listen to your body—when properly fed, lubricated, and exercised, it will perform wonderfully.

WATER

Room-temperature water consumed prior to a meal can stimulate the production of digestive enzymes. Water can even act as an appetite suppressant and actually help the body metabolize stored fats into usable energy.

Many people suffer from water retention and think that drinking water will add to the problem. Actually, the opposite is true. The more water we consume, the more we excrete. The body retains water when we are not taking in a sufficient amount to ensure survival. We can rectify the problem by simply drinking plenty of water.

I recommend drinking at least a half-gallon of distilled water daily. Carry a half-gallon container of water with you to work and back home again; don't go to bed until all the water in the container is consumed. This will help you become conscious of how much you need to drink. Always drink good-quality water, never from the tap (unless you have a reverse osmosis filter). I recommend distilled water, although many people prefer bottled spring water; the missing minerals in distilled water can be easily replaced with appropriate supplements. Most multivitamin/multimineral supplements provide a good balanced foundation of minerals in a bioavailable form. Review your supplements with a nutritionist or other knowledgeable health-care practitioner and ask her to suggest the type of water best suited for you.

EXERCISE

Most people find that regular exercise leads to regular bowel movements. This is because not only are the muscles conditioned during exercise, but the heart rate and circulation are also increased, along with metabolism and other body functions. Waste is moved throughout the intestines by a series of muscular contractions, gently forcing the stool out of the body. Muscle tone is an important factor in elimination. Exercise also enables the body to process and use the food more quickly, making it ready for elimination. Exercise is also a great stress reducer. Some exercises help strengthen the abdominal wall and increase oxygenation, both necessary for a healthy colon and a healthy body. Too much activity without time to rest and relax, however, can also hinder our bodily functions, including elimination.

Almost anyone can do some sort of exercise, regardless of his or her physical condition. Simply walking three times a week is wonderful to increase cardiovascular circulation, improve muscle tone, and help with digestion and elimination. If you're new to exercise, start by walking three minutes in one direction, then turn around and come back. Do this every other day. Walk at a comfortable pace, but try to gently increase your energy output and/or heart rate. The next week, walk four minutes in one direction, then turn around and come back. Each week increase the walking time by a minute. After a while, you may want to walk in the morning and in the evening. Build up to a thirty-minute walk each way. Using this method, even the most sedentary people can begin to develop a great exercise program that is effective but not threatening.

Ask your partner or a friend to join you, or use the quiet time to meditate and count all the good things in your life. Make a mental list of how you can share a smile that day. Breathe deeply. Walk with conviction. Know you are in charge of your health, and you are making a difference. Use this time to set your mental attitude for the rest of the day, or if you walk at night, reflect over the good fortunes, no matter how small, of the day that passed.

Exercise also brings with it the benefits of fresh air, the sunlight necessary for vitamin D and hormone production, or a view of the moon and stars at night. You may even meet some nice neighbors you didn't know you had. Give it a try! Consult your doctor before beginning any vigorous exercise program and proceed slowly. Exercise is also a great way to help reduce the effects of stress in our lives and promotes the elimination of toxins through perspiration and increased circulation.

DIET

The United States population is the most overfed, yet undernourished nation in the world. We consume more empty calories and processed foods than any other country. Even hospital food, chosen and prepared by so-called dietary specialists, falls short. Researchers from the State University of New York at Stony Brook and New York University reported in the *New England Journal of Medicine* that many of the facilities they studied failed to meet the guidelines set up by the U.S. Public Health Service as their national health goals for the year 2000. If the experts in the American Dietetic Association can't put together healthy meals in a hospital setting where good nutrition is essential to ensure quick recovery, how can we be expected to put together a meal for ourselves or our families to promote health and well-being? We are constantly bombarded with advertisements for newer, better, and quicker foods. We live in a time of stress and hurry. We are always looking for easier ways to provide nourishment that will satisfy our appetites but not require major preparation. The ads on TV are enticing, but our health is at stake. Don't be misled by Madison Avenue's message; it is geared to promote sales, not wellness. Everything we consume has an effect on our health, good or bad.

The Importance of Fiber

Our Standard American Diet (SAD) is sadly lacking in fiber. With sufficient intake of fresh fruits, vegetables, and whole grains, constipation would probably not be a problem.

There are basically seven types of fiber:

- Cellulose, an indigestible form of carbohydrate, is found in fruits and vegetables such as apples, celery, carrots, peas, and the outer shells of whole grains.
- Gums, resinlike substances, are found in plants such as guar.
- Lignans are found in Brazil nuts, potatoes, peas, and whole grains.
- Pectin, found in apples, bananas, citrus, carrots, and okra, is particularly helpful in reducing toxins.
- Hemicellulose, found in apples, bananas, beans, green leafy vegetables, cabbage, and whole grains, is another form of indigestible carbohydrate.
- Mucilages, sticky substances found in plants such as flaxseed, are good for lowering cholesterol and stabilizing blood sugar levels.
- Brans, found in the outer casings of whole grains, are good for helping to lower cholesterol.

As you can see, many of the same fruits and vegetables offer a variety of fiber types. Fiber sources should be varied to get the full protective benefit.

Fiber has many benefits in addition to healthy bowel movements. Hormone levels, like testosterone and estrogen, are diminished as the fiber soaks up the hormones, preventing them from recirculating back into the body. This important factor may be involved in protecting women from breast, ovarian, and uterine cancer, and men from testicular and prostate cancer. This same absorption process soaks up fats, particularly cholesterol, preventing it from getting back into the body. Heavy metals are also more easily excreted with a fiber-rich diet. Fiber scrapes the intestinal walls clean, preventing buildup and protecting against colon cancer.

Fiber helps us lose weight as the calories from fats are passed out of the body, rather than absorbed and stored as fat. Fiber slows down the digestive process so that the enzymes have a better opportunity to completely digest our meals. It also slows down the absorption of sugars, normalizing blood sugar levels.

With all those benefits, why don't we just take a fiber pill or powder? Fiber supplements come in a variety of forms, which seem to be a simple solution. The problem is that they may include unnatural additives, flavorings, colorings, and/or preservatives. Doctors often prescribe an orange-flavored powder that is added to water or juice to provide additional fiber, but potentially harmful additives and sweeteners give it its flavor and color.

A natural alternative is pure psyllium seed husks available at health food stores. This fiber is unadulterated, considerably cheaper than the flavored brands, and can be added to water or juice. It is less gas forming than wheat bran and gentle enough to be taken when there are digestive disorders such as irritable bowel syndrome. I suggest you start taking one-eighth to one-quarter of a teaspoon in a glass of water or diluted juice just before each meal, then gradually work up to a full teaspoon with each meal. You should immediately notice an increase in stool volume, then an increase in daily bowel movements. Alternatively, take the psyllium when you wake up and before bedtime. The same results may be achieved.

What about commercial fiber wafers? Alas, like Metamucil®, they, too, have additives and flavorings. A similar fiber intake can be achieved simply from eating high-fiber foods. Consider Scandinavian Bran Crisps (available in most health food stores) as a snack. A whole apple is loaded with fiber and vitamins, too.

If the diet is lacking fiber, supplements can be purchased in a health food store. I recommend a product called AbsorbaTrim by Fem Essentials. It contains chitosan, which is fiber derived from shellfish, but it also has ingredients that help stabilize blood sugar, suppress the appetite, and enhance the fat absorption of the fiber. Renew Life offers Fiber Smart, a hypoallergenic blend of fibers designed for internal cleansing. Yerba Prima has a variety of psyllium and mixed-fiber blends. One of the favorites of practitioners has been Sonne's #9, which is simply psyllium husk (*plantago ovato*). Many companies offer fiber in a variety of forms. Check with your health food store for what products meet your needs.

A basic healthy diet of unrefined high-fiber foods is the best way to prevent constipation or treat an existing problem. Unrefined means food in its most whole and natural state, not stripped of its outer shell (such as white bread and white rice), not bleached (such as white flour), not hydrogenated (such as margarine), and not colored, preserved, flavor enhanced, or enriched (like most convenience foods). A wide variety of foods in their natural state offers everything we need to be healthy, providing we prepare them in a healthy manner. An organically grown baked potato is a good source of fiber and full of nutrients, but if that same organically grown potato is made into French fries, deep-fried in hydrogenated oil, the nourishment value diminishes greatly.

Whole Grains

Unfortunately, the American public is involved in a love affair with white flour. Our children grew up watching balloon-covered loaves of bread representing the perfect food. In the not-too-distant past, we were encouraged to fill our plates with gooey, gluey pasta made of white flour. We all forgot that white flour and water are the ingredients in paper maché, that sticky substance that dries as hard as plaster and coats the delicate villi of the intestinal tract, thus reducing surface absorption area and preventing thorough cleansing of the digestive tract. The Food Guide Pyramid designed by the U.S. Department of Agriculture suggests eating six to eleven servings of breads, pastas, and cereals a day, regardless of whether they are from processed grains.

These nutrient-deficient foods must be avoided. They can be replaced with a variety of whole grains, including:

- Whole wheat in its pure, unadulterated form. Breads, crackers, pasta, even pretzels can all be found made with 100 percent whole-wheat flour. Be careful of misleading labels that say "wheat" bread on the front, when the small label on the back of the package reveals that enriched (processed) flour is the first and dominant ingredient; whole wheat may be third or fourth down the list. Be sure the first ingredient is whole wheat. Be aware that wheat contains gluten, however, and many people are sensitive to it. Although wheat bran may ease constipation in some individuals, it may cause it in others.

- Brown rice, which can be cooked and used like white rice in a variety of side dishes and added to soups and stews, is also used to make different forms of pasta and is available in flour and pancake mixes, cereals, breads, and cookies, providing a variety of products for those who want to avoid wheat. These products are gluten free and can be eaten by those with gluten sensitivities and celiac disease.

- Barley, another grain that contains gluten, is a wonderful addition to soups and pilafs, and is also available as flour and as both hot and cold cereals.

- Rye is added to white flour to make the traditional rye bread (most people mistakenly think that supermarket rye bread does not contain wheat). Cream of rye is a delicious hot cereal. Wheat-free rye bread is available in most health food stores; however, it also contains gluten.

- Millet is a tiny, round grain that can be toasted and then cooked like rice for a tasty side dish. It is available in cereals, can be added to soups, and can be incorporated into puddings and breads. Millet is gluten free.

- Quinoa (keen-wah) is similar to millet but with a stronger taste. It can be used as a side dish like rice. There are quinoa cereals and pastas, which usually include corn. Quinoa is gluten free.

- Kamut is an ancient form of wheat that has become quite popular. It belongs to the wheat family and should be avoided by those who require a wheat-free diet; it does contain gluten. It can be found in flour, cereals, and breads.

- Corn in the form of meal can be used in baking and cooking; polenta is a delicious side dish. Corn is usually mixed with wheat in foods such as cornbread and corn muffins, so read the label if you are sensitive to wheat. Corn pasta and fine corn flour, which can be used for baking, are available, as well as corn flakes and puffed corn cereals. Corn is gluten free.
- Oats are familiar to everyone as oatmeal or oat bran, but oat flour can also be purchased and used for baking. It makes great pancakes and mixes well with other flours. Oats do contain gluten.

Fruits and Vegetables

According to the American Dietetic Association, we should eat at least five servings of fruits and vegetables each day, including fruit juices. If one were to consume one glass of juice in the morning, a piece of fruit as an afternoon snack, a vegetable serving at lunch and dinner, and a small dinner salad, this would be accomplished. Sounds easy to do, but unfortunately, the majority of the population doesn't come close to meeting these recommendations, and if they do, they often include "vegetables" such as ketchup, French fries, and potato chips.

Whole fruits and vegetables can help relieve constipation, not only by their fiber content, but by their water content as well. Natural moisture from foods can help us meet our daily water intake requirements, since most people do not drink enough water on a regular basis. Another benefit of foods such as onion, garlic, Jerusalem artichoke, and asparagus is that they provide short-chain polysaccharides, such as fructooligosaccharides (FOS), which actually help keep the good intestinal flora flourishing. These "good" bacteria keep "bad" bacteria in check.

Whole, fresh fruits (not juices) and fresh vegetables, taken in proper amounts, provide plenty of fiber to keep the bowels moving. In fact, recent guidelines suggest five to nine servings of fruits and vegetables daily to prevent cancer. The fiber in fresh fruit slows down sugar absorption, so that blood sugar doesn't rise as fast as it does with fruit juice. High-fiber foods also take longer to digest, so we are not as hungry. Steamed vegetables with a little flaxseed oil added to give a rich, buttery taste provide a nutritious addition to any meal. Be creative with your vegetable choices; don't eat the same ones all the time. Use spices and condiments to brighten the taste.

I couldn't get my kids to eat broccoli until I realized that a little flax oil and some whole-grain, seasoned bread crumbs could transform broccoli into one of their favorite dishes. My older daughter hated cooked carrots until I tried a recipe of sautéed carrots in tamari with strips of kombu (seaweed) added. Now she begs me to make it. One of my children's favorite snacks is raw red pepper, eaten alone or dipped in hummus. They love to take this to school in their lunchboxes. Soups and stews are wonderful ways to get vegetables into you and your kids. They are easy to make; they can be prepared in advance and frozen for future use or cooked slowly in a crockpot. A little planning is needed, but it can be done. See pages 36 to 37 for my family's favorite recipes.

Here are some other produce tips. When I come home from the grocery with a large amount of produce, I clean out the kitchen sink and fill it with clean water and a little bleach (a teaspoon of bleach to 2 gallons of clean water). Take the damaged outer leaves off the lettuces and place all the produce in the water for a good fifteen to twenty minutes. This kills any bacteria that may be on the produce. Some people believe that organically grown produce need not be carefully washed. This is untrue. Consider that organic farming is done with natural manure and compost. Very often bacteria grow, contributing to the ecocycle, but this should not be consumed. Besides, handling and packing may bring more germs. Washing produce in this manner will also give it moisture to keep it fresh and supple. Drain and whisk leafy greens dry; wrap in a clean dish towel and place in a plastic bag. Your greens will remain fresh and crisp for at least five days.

Buying fresh vegetables is always better than buying canned. In fact, canned foods should be avoided as much as possible to prevent aluminum and sodium buildup in the body. Frozen is the next best choice, but not always available in organically grown form (except in larger health food grocery stores). I take advantage of the sales on organic produce at the health food stores. I bring some distilled or mineral water (never tap water) to a boil, add a little seasoning, and place the cleaned vegetables in for just one minute. I am careful to use a timer, as overcooking will yield mushy veggies. After boiling for one minute, I drain the blanched vegetables in a colander and run cold water over them to stop the cooking process. Then I package the vegetables in portioned containers and freeze. This is an inexpensive way to have my organic vegetables, cleaned and ready to use in a short time. I prepare the vegetables on the weekend when time isn't a factor. This is also a great time to make and freeze vegetable soups and stews. With a little planning and creativity, eating vegetables can be simple and delicious.

Vegetables, fruits, and grains that should be increased in or added to your diet include cabbage, carrots, beans, okra, kale, peas, sweet potatoes, apples, pears, citrus fruits, raisins, figs, flaxseed, dark green lettuces, whole grains, brown rice, and just about any fresh fruit or vegetable you prefer. Be creative in preparation and combinations. Experiment with spices and different types of vegetables. Become adventurous. Try something new each week. Encourage your family, especially your children, to taste different vegetables and exotic fruits. My daughters enjoy fruits such as pomegranate, kumquat, carambola, and kiwi. Try using rutabaga or malanga (a root vegetable similar to yucca and used by many Latin Americans). Invest in some good vegetarian cookbooks. Use fruits in smoothies and shakes. Make your own applesauce or other fruit sauce. Use fruit as a reward for younger children so that they learn to appreciate and desire it instead of sweets. Have lots of cut-up vegetables available in the refrigerator for snacks. Many stores offer washed and cleaned organic baby carrots. Try different ethnic restaurants such as Mexican, Italian, or Chinese; they often prepare native fruits and vegetables in a variety of ways.

Take your time; don't make a drastic transition as the shock may thwart your efforts. Plan ahead. Make a list of what you want to buy and what meals you have in mind for the week. This will help discourage you from grabbing a fast-food substitute. Avoid processed foods. They tend to be void of nutrition and high in unhealthy additives. Try to eat food in its most natural form.

In addition to adding a variety of grains, fruits, and vegetables to your diet, try some new and exotic foods such as seaweed, seeds, nuts, and tofu. Once you get past the image of that greenish-brown mass that washes ashore, you will find that seaweed is a delicious and nutritious addition to the diet. I add kombu to all of my cooked beans and most of my soups. This wide, dark seaweed adds a wonderful flavor, contributes lots of vitamins and minerals, and makes the meal more digestible. My daughters really enjoy a carrot kombu sauté (see recipes on page 36). Nori is the dark, paper-thin squares in which sushi is rolled. Nori is great when toasted and sprinkled on top of a salad or baked potato. Kelp is easily added to the diet; it comes in a shaker and can be sprinkled on just about any dish. Hijiki and aramé have a stronger flavor. Go to a good health food or Japanese restaurant and taste these sea vegetables properly prepared before you try preparing them yourself. They make wonderful salads and additions to brown rice.

Seeds

Seeds may conjure up images of bird food, but this often-overlooked food is a wonderful source of protein and nutrients. Flaxseed is mucilaginous and helps bowel motility; it also has an abundant supply of essential fatty acids that are important to good health. I always add ground flaxseeds to oatmeal or any cooked cereal. I also adore the flavor of flax-seed sprinkled into the uncooked side of a rice pancake as it sizzles on the griddle. Be aware that a stray seed may pop if left directly on the pan. Flaxseed can be ground in a coffee grinder and added to just about any food. The grinding helps release many omega-3 fatty acids, the essential oil rarely found in plants that is also found in salmon and other fatty cold-water fish. It is advisable to grind just what you will use to prevent the released oils from turning rancid. Flaxseed soaked in water for several hours and removed results in a thick liquid substance that can be used as an egg replacement in recipes; this is a boon for those who are sensitive to eggs.

Sunflower seeds are a great source of omega-6 fatty acids and can be easily sprinkled on cereals, added to baked goods for a nutritious crunch, or simply eaten out of hand. Sesame seeds are a good source of calcium and have a wonderful flavor. A traditional Italian holiday treat is a butter cookie rolled in sesame seeds. Ground sesame seeds produce tahini, the tasty ingredient in hummus and salad dressings. Sesame seeds also are great as a coating for chicken or simply sprinkled over a salad. Pumpkin seeds are a good source of zinc and are a great support for the prostate. Baked fish coated with chopped pumpkin seeds and mango salsa is a delectable dish. Poppy seeds give a wonderful flavor to fresh whole-grain rolls. Consumption of too many poppy seeds, however, cause a positive result on a drug test (poppy is the original source of opium).

Nuts

Nuts are often taken for granted as the salted treat we serve at a party, but they are a great source of nutrients and necessary good oils. Nuts can be added to salads, mixed with fruit or whole-grain cereals, or added to homemade breads, muffins, and cookies. They can be ground and mixed with ground meat to add flavor and reduce animal fat intake, or they can be soaked in water overnight and made into a milk substitute for those with milk sensitivity. Nuts can be made into the most wonderful butters. Instead of peanut butter, try pistachio, almond, hazelnut, or cashew butter. Peanuts are probably the worst choice for nuts, as many people are highly allergic to them. Peanuts also often contain a mold that can trigger negative reactions in the body, and they are poorly digested. Try a gradual inclusion of other nuts into your diet.

Tofu

Tofu as well as soy in general have been getting quite a lot of good press lately since the media finally realized what we in the alternative health profession have been saying all along about the benefits of soy. Soy products (especially tofu) are not only more nutritious than meat and animal products but also actually help prevent disease, including hormone-related cancers. Tofu is soybean curd that is shaped into a white block. It is tasteless, but can easily be made to taste like whatever you add to it. It is high in protein, can be low in fat, and is a better source of calcium than milk. If blended with fruit juice and fresh fruit, it makes a wonderful high-protein shake for a quick breakfast. Marinated and grilled, it makes a tasty meat substitute. You can bake with it, make creamy puddings and desserts, add it to stir-fries instead of chicken or meat, or crumble it into a tasty scrambled egg substitute.

Food Sensitivities

No discussion of diet would be complete without addressing food sensitivities. Most people think that runny nose, watery eyes, and sneezing are the only symptoms of food sensitivities, but reactions could also include headache, back and joint aches, gas, diarrhea, and constipation. Food sensitivities are often the result of eating too much of our favorite foods, the ones we consume on a frequent or daily basis. True food allergy, however, causes an immediate reaction, such as swelling of the throat and tongue after eating strawberries, shellfish, or peanuts, which can result in anaphylactic shock. This is a true medical emergency; therefore, these substances must always be avoided at all costs by susceptible individuals.

Food sensitivities result in much milder symptoms that may occur immediately or even days after the offending food is ingested. Typically, these are foods that we most often eat, such as wheat, corn, dairy, sugar, and soy. Many times food sensitivities result from increased gut permeability, or "leaky gut" syndrome when partially digested food particles pass through the digestive lumen into the bloodstream. This is a result of poor eating habits, improper digestion, and over-the-counter or prescription medications. The body cannot identify these foods in the partially digested form, so it reacts as if a foreign invader arrived, responding with distress in the respiratory, gastrointestinal, or musculoskeletal systems.

By identifying and temporarily eliminating these foods, one may eventually be able to eat them again on a rotation basis, providing intestinal integrity is restored and the digestive process is enhanced. There are several ways for health practitioners to identify food sensitivities, but a simple method to determine your own sensitivities is by recording your pulse before and after eating the questionable food. A normal resting pulse rate is fifty-five to seventy beats per minute. If your pulse rate increases by more than ten beats per minute after eating the selected food, chances are you are sensitive to it. Eliminate that particular food from your diet for about three weeks while monitoring any changes in symptoms, then eat the offending food in its simplest form and notice if your symptoms reoccur. Food elimination gives the body a chance to recover, and supplements can help restore the gut integrity. Rotating all foods at least every other day helps the body cope with sensitivities. I recommend keeping a daily food diary.

Some practitioners believe that food sensitivities and the way each individual digests and processes food are not only related but may be the underlying cause of all disease. This theory has even been the foundation of some successful weight-loss programs. It's worth a try; you may feel better eliminating some common foods from your daily diet. And you may see a dramatic difference in your bowel habits. Dairy foods and wheat are common culprits in constipation.

Buy Organic Whenever Possible
Organically grown food is produced in fields that have been unexposed to chemicals and fertilizers for at least seven years. These crops are naturally fertilized, usually in composted soil, and not sprayed with pesticides. It may be more expensive to put ladybugs in the fields to keep the pests down, but it is a small price to pay to keep the dangerous toxins out of our food supply. These organically grown plants are not picked before their time or gassed to stimulate ripening. They are not waxed or irradiated. They are not genetically engineered to produce more yield or to enable a machine to pick them. They are in the purest form, the way nature intended.

Perhaps the most important benefit is that these foods are significantly higher in nutrition than those that are commercially grown. An organically grown tomato has 40 percent more magnesium in it than a commercially grown tomato, not to mention significantly better taste. Most of today's crops are lacking in minerals such as selenium and magnesium as the soil has been depleted due to overuse. The ground is not set aside to lie fallow and replenish itself. It is chemically altered to replace some of the nutrients that have leeched out of the soil, but man can never do better than nature.

Organic produce often does cost more. This is because each crop has a smaller yield and shorter shelf life, but it is worth the price. Most grocery stores are adding organic sections to their produce departments. Ask your produce manager to consider carrying organically grown food. As the demand increases, availability will also increase. Start with just a single item, perhaps carrots. Notice the difference in taste, then gradually make the switch item by item. You will learn to tell the difference and your body will thank you.

Food Combining

Food combining can be very important to the digestive system. The typical American meal combines protein and carbohydrates, whether it is meat and potatoes, a tuna sandwich, spaghetti and meatballs, peanut butter and jelly, or pepperoni pizza. Yet different enzymes are required to break down protein and carbohydrate and different levels of acidity in the digestive tract. When both are consumed at the same time, neither one is properly digested, resulting in fermentation and gas. Even though breaking old habits is difficult to do, it is really important to avoid mixing protein and carbohydrates in the same meal as much as possible. With a little effort, you will find that food combining is not as difficult as you imagined.

In addition, eat fruits alone—at least two hours before or after a meal. The reason for this is that fruits are digested very rapidly and move out of the stomach in a short time so they can be further broken down in the small intestine. If you combine fruits with other foods, it delays their time in the stomach and hinders digestion. I recommend three fresh, whole, organic (if possible) fruits a day, eaten between meals as snacks. For example, have a fruit between breakfast and lunch, in the afternoon between lunch and dinner, and before bedtime. This helps increase fiber intake, provides healthful phytonutrients, and helps keep blood sugar levels from dropping too low. Fruit is also a low-calorie snack that satisfies the sweet tooth. Fruit juice is no substitute for fresh fruit. It takes several oranges to produce a glass of orange juice. That's a lot of sugar without the fiber to slow down its absorption. It is far better to eat the whole fruit than simply the juice.

MY FAVORITE RECIPES

Tofu Fruit Shake
3 oz. silken tofu

1 frozen banana

3–4 frozen strawberries

4 oz. unsweetened apple juice

Blend until well mixed and enjoy.

Kombu Carrots
1 tbs. olive oil

3 thin carrots, sliced

1 tbs. tamari

1 strip of kombu, rinsed and
soaked for 15 minutes, then cut
into ½″ strips

Heat oil in skillet and stir-fry carrot slices until soft. Add tamari and kombu (include some of the water it was soaked in). Simmer for 15 minutes and serve.

Oatmeal Flaxseed Muffins
2 cups of rolled oats

2 cups oat bran

2 tsp. baking powder

2 eggs, beaten

1 cup apple juice

¼ cup maple syrup

3 tbs. flaxseeds

4 apples, diced

⅓ cup dried cranberries

Combine dry ingredients. Combine wet ingredients in separate bowl. Mix both together with seeds and fruit. Pour into paper-lined muffin tins. Preheat oven to 350°. Bake for 25 to 30 minutes.

Kale and Carrot Soup
1 tbs. olive oil

1 onion, diced

2 cloves garlic

3 stalks celery, sliced

4 shiitake mushrooms (fresh or
dried)

1 small piece of ginger, grated

1 gallon water

2 tbs. vegetable broth powder

1 tbs. Bragg Liquid Aminos

1 tsp. turmeric

1 tsp. salt

Black pepper to taste

4 potatoes

5 carrots

1 bunch fresh kale, washed and cut
off the main vein

Dash of raw unfiltered apple cider
vinegar (optional)

Place oil in a large soup pot, and sauté onions, garlic, celery, mushrooms, and fresh ginger until tender. Add water and bring to a boil. Mix in vegetable broth powder and seasonings.

Add potatoes, carrots, and kale. Reduce heat and simmer until tender.

Escarole Bean Soup

1 tbs. olive oil
8 cloves garlic, minced
1 gallon pure water
12 oz. great northern beans, soaked
   overnight, rinsed, and drained
1 head green cabbage, chopped
1 stalk kombu (sea vegetable)
1 cup parsley, chopped

1 tsp. fennel seeds
8–10 leaves fresh basil, chopped
1 tsp. crushed red pepper (optional)
2 large heads escarole, chopped
1 tbs. Bragg Liquid Aminos
1 tbs. salt
Black pepper to taste

Place oil in a large soup pot, and sauté garlic until tender. Add water and bring to a boil. Add beans, cabbage, kombu, parsley, fennel seeds, basil, and red pepper. After it boils again, reduce heat and simmer uncovered for 90 minutes. Be sure to stir frequently. Add escarole, liquid aminos, salt, and black pepper and continue cooking 1 hour or until beans are tender.

Broccoli with Bread Crumbs

1 large head of organic broccoli,
   washed and cut into spears
3 tbs. of flaxseed oil

2 tbs. Jaclyn's Bread Crumbs mixed
   with salt, pepper, and garlic to taste

Steam broccoli until tender (but not overcooked). Drizzle oil over broccoli, cover with bread-crumb mixture, and gently stir. Serve warm.

Hummus

⅓ cup tahini
1 cup cooked garbanzo beans
   (chick peas)
1 clove garlic

1½ tbs. tamari
2 tbs. fresh-squeezed lemon juice
Dash of paprika

Blend all ingredients in a food processor until smooth and creamy. Serve with whole-grain pita bread wedges, as a dip with raw vegetables, or in a sandwich with alfalfa sprouts and sliced tomato.

Some ways to promote a healthy intestinal environment as well as assure good digestion and nutrient absorption are discussed in the following sections.

DIGESTIVE ENZYMES

The foods we eat must be broken down into smaller particles before the nutrients can be digested and absorbed. Thus, even if one consumes a perfectly healthy diet, the body may still be lacking in essential nutrients if digestion is faulty. Although the body produces enzymes to help digestion, certain enzymes are found right in the food we eat when it is consumed in its most natural and unprocessed form. When our diet consists of mostly refined, processed foods, the body must work harder to supply itself with needed nourishment. This extra effort to produce enzymes and digest food uses precious energy that could be well spent on other bodily functions such as healing, detoxing, cell repair, and regeneration. Thus, repetitive malabsorption can lead to many chronic diseases. This is another good reason to eat wholesome, unadulterated foods.

Digestion starts in the mouth and continues in the stomach and on into the small intestine. We've all felt our mouths water at the idea of a great meal, which proves that digestive juices can start to flow even before we begin eating. Just the thought, sight, or smell of food can signal the stomach to get ready to eat. This external stimulation sends a message to the hypothalamus in the brain that food is on the way. The hypothalamus then sends a signal down to the stomach glands to let the juices flow. When the food enters the stomach, the enzymes are there to greet it. If the food is not soon ingested, we get that gnawing pain that we call hunger. Alcohol and stress, however, can also get these juices flowing, often without any food to follow. The highly acidic gastric secretions soon begin to eat away at the mucosal lining of the stomach itself, eventually forming an ulcer.

Digestion and absorption continue in different stages throughout the gastrointestinal tract, providing us with the needed nutrients to not only sustain life but to function at our maximum capacity (providing that quality food is ingested). Very often we eat on the run, make poor food choices, dilute our enzymes with sweetened drinks, and improperly combine our food (eating protein and carbohydrates together). This hinders the body's natural ability to transform food into a usable form. If these habits are not corrected, health problems can occur, and we may need a little help from enzyme supplements. The following digestive enzymes can be easily added to the meal at the time of ingestion to assure that the body has the tools to break down food and absorb its nourishment.

Hydrochloric Acid (HCl)

Hydrochloric acid (usually with pepsin), available as a capsule or tablet, is an important supplement for those with low HCl levels in the stomach. Indications of low stomach acid are:

- Gas and belching after a meal
- Needing to unbutton your pants even after consuming small amounts of food
- Skin disorders such as psoriasis or rosacea
- Nails that split and peel in layers
- Anemia
- A burning sensation in your stomach after you eat
- Frequent yeast infections
- Rashes under the arm and in the groin

- Athlete's foot
- Halitosis

The sure way to determine *hypochlorhydria* (low stomach acid) is to have your physician test you with a tiny transmitter that measures the actual stomach acidity. If acid is low, adding supplements may be a simple solution. One easy way to test if supplementing with HCl is right for you is to place a teaspoon of raw, unfiltered apple cider vinegar into 4 ounces of pure water and drink it after a meal. *Important:* Have baking soda available before trying this test, and do not try it at all if you have been diagnosed with ulcers. Be sure to rinse your mouth out afterwards as the vinegar can eat away at your tooth enamel. You should feel the sensation of the vinegar going down your throat and into your stomach, but there may be a deep burning in your stomach. If there is a painful burning, take a teaspoon of baking soda mixed with 4 ounces of water. This will immediately neutralize the acid and relieve the pain. If you find relief with the apple cider vinegar, you may be a candidate for supplemental HCl. If you find that the vinegar caused discomfort, you may have too much stomach acid and should *not* take HCl, but consider supplemental enzymes that work further down the intestinal tract.

Pancreatin

Pancreatin is a protein-digesting enzyme produced in the pancreas; it can be purchased in supplemental form. Signs of pancreatic dysfunction include gas, bloating, some food sensitivities, and signs of undigested food and/or fat in the stool. It can also manifest as low blood sugar, yeast infections, or parasitic infections. Pancreatin works best in an alkaline environment, so purchase a supplement that is enteric coated (this is a protective coating added to protect the enzyme from the harsh stomach acid so it will be released in the alkaline environment of the small intestine). This supplement, unlike HCl, can be taken without food to help chronic degenerative diseases.

Lactase

Lactase is the enzyme that helps break down the sugars (lactose) found in milk. It is available in pill form and is sometimes added directly to bottled milk for those who are lactose intolerant. People with lactose intolerance have immediate stomach upset after ingesting dairy-containing foods. The usual manifestation is gas and diarrhea. Milk consists of very large protein molecules and is difficult to digest for most people. I believe milk is best avoided, but if you do consume dairy products, you may want to consider a lactase supplement.

Bromelain

Bromelain is the enzyme found in fresh pineapple that causes your tongue to burn after too much is consumed. It breaks down protein, and your tongue tingles because your taste buds have been exposed to too much at one time. Pineapple pickers sometimes find that their fingerprints are slowly eaten away by the constant exposure of their hands to pineapple juice. But this potent enzyme activity is wonderful not only for aiding digestion but also for reducing inflammation. In fact, if it is taken on an empty stomach after an injury or surgery, it will help eat away any extravasated blood (bruising or black and blue marks) or torn tissue.

Papain

Papain is another plant enzyme, found in papaya, which, like bromelain, aids in protein digestion. Papain is sometimes injected into the ruptured disks of those with back injuries to eat away the cartilaginous disks and thus avoid back surgery. This potent enzyme is great for ridding the walls of the intestines of dead, encrusted waste material. It, too, can be used without food to reduce inflamation, but when taken with a meal, it can help digestion.

Ginger

Ginger is one of my favorite herbs as it is so versatile. It helps digest protein and can also help to heal ulcers, soothe

the stomach, relieve nausea and vomiting, and kill parasites. It helps to tone the heart, yet it stimulates liver function so that cholesterol can be converted into bile to aid digestion. I always carry a bottle of liquid ginger extract in my car for carsickness and the occasional upset stomach. A liquid extract is recommended to help the digestion of those who cannot swallow pills.

Combination Enzymes

Combination digestive enzymes are also available at health food stores. They usually include a variety of many of the previously discussed enzymes. This is usually the safest way to begin taking enzymes as they enhance the total digestive process while not requiring the diagnosis of specific enzyme deficiency. For those who are vegetarian, these enzyme complexes are available in a totally vegetarian tablet. If enzyme deficiency is your problem, you will shortly notice a reduction of symptoms such as gas and bloating. You will feel less full after a meal and may experience a reduction of abdominal discomfort. Remember this is not a panacea, but a way to encourage more complete digestion, which will lead to more nutrient absorption and better colon health.

REMOVING PARASITES

Parasites are often only associated with Third World countries where diarrhea can be life threatening. The truth is, however, that there are hundreds of thousands of Americans living with over 130 types of parasites. Contracting a parasite is easy to do with today's contaminated water supply, international travel, sexual freedom, and exposure to domestic animals. Frequently, diarrhea and malabsorption occur when there is a parasite infestation, but it can also be the cause of constipation. (As previously mentioned, Great Smokies Lab offers the best testing in their Comprehensive Digestive Stool Analysis.) Large parasites such as tapeworms and roundworms can block the common bile duct, hindering biliary flow and digestion, and can also obstruct the intestines themselves, causing constipation and pain.

Herbs such as garlic, grapefruit seed extract, black walnut, and wormwood are useful for ridding the body of parasites. A severe infestation should be handled by your health-care professional. For general maintenance, there are products available that not only detox the colon but kill yeast and parasites as well. I recommend that my clients do a "preventive cleaning" once a year to maintain good colon health. I suggest prepared programs such as Paragone by Renew Life, which helps kill parasites, cleans the colon, supports liver cleansing, and restores gut flora. This is available at your health food store. These prepared combinations have the advantage of killing several types of parasites. Individual remedies may work on some but not others and are therefore best used after parasitology tests are done.

PROBIOTICS

Probiotics are the good bacteria residing in the intestinal tract. Most of us are familiar with acidophilus, found mostly in the small intestine, and bifidobacteria, found mostly in the colon, but there are other types of less widely known, but still important, gut flora. There should be approximately 4 pounds of good bacteria in each adult individual, but this isn't always the case. Many times good bacteria are destroyed by antibiotics, steroids, stress, diet, and constipation. Babies delivered by Cesarean section, as well as formula-fed babies, are known to have fewer numbers of good gut flora. Lack of probiotics compromises our health by not allowing us to digest our food or absorb the nutrients of the food we ingest. It also allows the proliferation of "bad" bacteria and yeast, hinders our elimination, and affects our immune systems.

In 1988, the U.S. Surgeon General stated, "Normal microbial flora provide a passive mechanism to prevent infection." They do this by crowding out the harmful bacteria, as well as their toxic by-products, and by producing acids such as formic acid, lactic acid, and acetic acid, making an unsuitable environment for pathogenic bacteria. Good gut flora help the body manufacture and utilize B vitamins, folic acid, and vitamins A and K. These friendly critters produce lactic acid, which helps us absorb copper, calcium, iron, magnesium, and manganese. They help build our resistance to food poisoning, as well as stimulate the production of defensive immune cells. Friendly flora help protect us from harmful pollution in the environment and also have antitumor effects. Good gut flora are also involved in maintaining normal serum cholesterol and triglyceride levels. They help break down bile acids remaining from the digestive process. They help regulate normal bowel movements, promoting regularity, and can help prevent vaginal yeast infections, along with other fungal infections.

Most people think that friendly bacteria are easily supplied by eating yogurt. This is true if you select the right yogurt; however, most of the yogurts found in the grocery stores have very low levels of live flora, and contain too many sweeteners, emulsifiers, and additives to do much good. The organic yogurt found in your health food store is less processed and higher in flora than the brands found in most supermarkets. Probiotics are also found in sauerkraut, miso, tempeh, and tamari. Green tea, ginseng, Jerusalem artichoke, and bananas all help the proliferation of good bacteria; the latter two are high in FOS, which promote rapid reproduction of good bacteria. Friendly flora can be purchased in your health food store. Select from those kept in the refrigerator, which helps to maintain their viability. Also check the potency and the kinds of bacteria in each product. Different products provide different numbers of bacteria. They should number in the billions.

I recommend a powder such as Jarrodophilis, DDS, or Vital Life for easy administration, high potency, and the fact that it comes with FOS already in it. Nutrition Now and Renew Life have coated flora products that require no refrigeration. This makes for easier traveling. Some products should not be taken with food, while the action of others is enhanced when taken with food. Be sure to check the label for instructions. Be aware that these live bacteria have a limited life span in the jar. Do not keep them in your refrigerator for a year or two. Buy what you will use in a short time; then buy fresh again. Ask your health-care practitioner to recommend a specific product to meet your needs.

FOS

FOS (fructooligosaccharides) increases the proliferation of probiotics in your gut. FOS is a sugar with a long molecular structure, which accounts for its sweet taste. But this sugar is not readily broken down and absorbed into the body. Instead, it passes intact through the digestive tract where it feeds the good bacteria and encourages their reproduction. The good news is that FOS adds its sweetness with minimal caloric absorption. It does not have a negative effect on diabetics or hypoglycemics; in fact, it may actually help them.

Presently, Japan has over five hundred products containing FOS such as soft drinks, candies, cereals, sweeteners, and desserts. By adding FOS, some of the sucrose (table sugar) can be reduced as well as calories. FOS is naturally found in foods such as garlic, honey, brown sugar, bananas, onions, soy, barley, tomatoes, and Jerusalem artichokes. Although it is found in these foods, there is actually too little to be of major benefit. I recommend using it supplementally in pill form or in a powder that can be sprinkled on food. One gram of FOS added to the daily diet can help increase good gut flora by a factor of five. Keep in mind that if your intestines are not in the best of health, you may want to start with a really small amount, then gradually build up to one-fourth of a teaspoon to avoid the production of gas. Hopefully, we will also have it added to our foods soon, as it is in Japan.

NATURAL ASSISTANCE FOR CONSTIPATION

Everyone will experience constipation at one time or another. The occasional natural remedy will do no harm. Problems occur when these remedies become habitual. Please remember that these are once-in-awhile remedies. Diet, exercise, and water are the everyday foundation of good bowel habits.

MAGNESIUM

Seventy percent of the approximate 1 ounce of magnesium found in the body is located in the teeth and bones. The most important functions of this mineral, however, are due to the remaining 30 percent, which activates many enzymes and controls a number of functions within the cells. It is involved with protein formation, the storage and release of energy, and the function and formation of DNA, as well as muscle relaxation and the proper utilization of calcium. Many people notice an increase in energy after taking magnesium for a week or so. This is because magnesium is necessary for the production of ATP (energy) in each cell. If each cell has a higher energy output, then the organism will have more energy at its disposal.

Magnesium is also very important in carbohydrate metabolism. People with a lower ratio of magnesium to calcium tend to have more blood sugar problems. Most hypoglycemics suffer from a lack of high-magnesium foods in their diets. Many people who fall asleep easily but awaken after a few hours do so because of a blood sugar problem; this usually improves with magnesium supplementation at dinner or bedtime.

Arthritis and kidney stones are often prevented by adequate magnesium intake. A five-year study at Boston University indicated that magnesium supplementation dramatically reduced the incidence of kidney stone formation. Similarly, magnesium prevents the deposition of calcium on the joints (arthritis). The relaxation effect that magnesium has on muscles makes it helpful in dealing with most muscle cramps and spasms. Menstrual cramps are contractions of the uterine muscle. As the muscle relaxes, the cramps lessen. Many good PMS formulas contain significant amounts of magnesium. The same is also true of those who suffer from leg cramps and other muscle pain. Are you eating enough green veggies? They are the best source of magnesium.

Constipation is often relieved with added magnesium. We all remember being given Milk of Magnesia or M.O. (magnesium oxide) when we were children. Citrate of magnesia is often given before a hospital procedure. Simply put, magnesium encourages bowel evacuation. This is a well-known fact. If our diets provided a sufficient supply of magnesium, however, we wouldn't need to supplement with this crucial mineral. Most people are magnesium deficient because their diets lack enough green leafy vegetables. This dietary deficiency can result in myriad complications, including increased blood pressure, muscle spasms, low blood sugar, lack of energy, poor calcium utilization, insomnia, and constipation.

It has been said that if everyone took a regular magnesium supplement, we would reduce our hospitalizations by 50 percent. I have had wonderful results recommending magnesium glycinate or magnesium aspartate to my clients. My sister, who suffers from high blood pressure, has had a problem with constipation for many years, so severe that she was scheduled to have surgery on the sigmoid-rectal area. Just days before the appointed surgery date, I convinced her to try magnesium. The results were so impressive that she canceled the surgery. It has been two years since she began taking a daily magnesium supplement, and not only is her blood pressure lower than it has ever been, she still has no problems with irregularity. Her doctor is pleased, and she saved her insurance company several thousand dollars.

One should not rely on magnesium or any other substance, herb, or laxative for daily bowel movements, however. Studies have indicated that magnesium abuse can be as detrimental to health as other types of laxatives used in excess. In fact, magnesium-induced diarrhea is more difficult to identify than laxative abuse, since magnesium is a component of body fluids and more difficult to detect. If your body is deficient in magnesium, though, supplementing it may be all you need to regulate your colon. Talk to your health-care practitioner to determine this. Let him or her assist you in making the decision. A simple tissue analysis can identify not only your mineral levels but also the ratios of each to the others.

A word of caution: Some medications require that you avoid magnesium supplementation. Please check with your physician first, then consult your licensed nutrition counselor or health-care practitioner to determine the type of magnesium and the dose that are best suited to your needs.

TOILET STOOLS

Toilet stools are relatively new on the natural health scene, although the technique of squatting to defecate has been around since the beginning of mankind. These convenient little stools sit at the foot of your toilet and can slide underneath and out of the way when not in use. When the user rests his or her feet on the stool, bringing the knees closer to the body, it puts the body in a sort of squatting position while sitting on the toilet. Squatting is nature's way of assuring a more natural and complete elimination. When we are in the usual sitting position on the toilet, the rectoanal angle of the intestinal tract is partially closed, requiring more effort to expel wastes. By raising the knees we straighten this angle, allowing a more opened passage out of the body. Also, the pressure of the legs against the lower abdomen helps the exertion of elimination; some researchers report that in the squatting position, one to several ounces more of waste is eliminated. This reduces the likelihood of hemorrhoids, eases elimination, and lowers the strain on the cardiovascular system.

I must admit that I was skeptical until I got a "Life Step" toilet stool. It truly feels better to eliminate with your feet up. At first you might feel awkward sitting on the toilet with your feet elevated, but you will quickly adjust and reap the benefits. You might try for yourself by using a low stool. The only drawback with a makeshift stool is that it tends to get in the way when not in use. Most bathrooms are small and it makes it difficult to navigate at night. The Life Step is made to wrap around the base of your toilet when not in use, so it's safe, convenient, and easy to clean. It is manufactured by Renew Life and is available in larger health food stores or by calling 1-800-830-4778 to find the retailer nearest you. It's worth the effort.

Whichever method you choose, take steps to reduce the stress on your body and help it work better for you.

HERBAL REMEDIES

According to Humberto Santillo, in his book *Natural Healing with Herbs*, there are three types of bowel-stimulating herbs: aperients, laxatives, and purgatives.

Aperients are slow acting and can be safely taken regularly. They include foods such as olive or flaxseed oil, dried fruits (figs, prunes, and raisins), seeds (chia, psyllium, and flax), seaweed (agar agar or kanten), turkey, rhubarb, and licorice root.

Laxatives stimulate bowel evacuation more quickly than aperients and should not be used on a daily basis but only to help the body empty, detoxify, and heal occasionally. These include the herbs aloe vera, cascara sagrada, wahoo bark, dandelion root (when the liver is involved), and rhubarb, which contains oxalic acid and should be avoided by those who have kidney stones, arthritis, and gout. Santillo says that during a fever these herbs will help cool the body by eliminating the heat-holding stool from the intestines (an alternative to an enema). Laxatives are typically taken at bedtime and can be taken singly or combined. They can cause gas and cramping, so be careful.

Purgatives act quickly and are known to drain energy from the body. Santillo includes American mandrake root, jalap, castor oil, buckthorn bark, and senna in his list of purgatives. These should not be used by anyone with hemorrhoids, dropped bladder or uterus, intestinal bleeding, or vomiting. These should also be avoided if there is abdominal pain, especially in the area of the appendix. Make sure you have a strong constitution before trying these purgatives, and use them only with the guidance of a health professional. Some practitioners feel that purgatives are dangerous and should not be used at all.

For children, Santillo recommends 1 ounce of raspberry leaves mixed with 1½ ounces of flaxseed. Pour 1 quart of boiling water over the herbs and seeds and let them steep for one-half hour; strain and administer 2 tablespoons three times a day.

Herbalist Gail Ulrich recommends 10 drops of yellow dock tincture in a little water to gently stimulate the liver, which in turn stimulates action. Some people may need a dropperful of tincture or twice-a-day application to get things moving again. Colon therapist Brenda Watson has formulated a wonderful two-part colon-cleansing product called "Cleanse Smart" by Renew Life. Part I is taken in the morning to cleanse the organs; Part II is taken in the evening and contains eight natural compounds (magnesium hydroxide, cape aloe, rhubarb root, slippery elm bark, marshmallow root, fennel seed, gingerroot, and triphala). Ayurvedic medicine recommends triphala, which is a combination of the dried groundfruit of three East Indian trees, to stimulate peristaltic contractions. I've recommended this product after a colon-cleansing regimen, particularly after someone had been habitually abusing laxatives. It helps encourage the muscles to begin working again. Flaxseed tea also works well and is simple to make. Simply boil a teaspoon of flaxseed in 1½ cups of water for ten minutes.

There are some ancient remedies for constipation that have been passed down for generations throughout different cultures.

- Hawaiians traditionally use watermelon pulp.
- The Dutch recommend simmering six cloves in 2 tablespoons of water for about one minute, then add cold water, steep for ten minutes, strain, and drink each day.
- German tribes mixed a tablespoon of honey into a little warm water, added a glass of cold water, and drank this first thing in the morning.
- Traditional Chinese medicine (TCM) maintains that fever, strength, dryness, and/or coagulation cause constipation. Depending on the pattern of symptoms, TCM practitioners may recommend rhubarb, cinnamon, or peony.

Constipation is a sign that there is something out of balance. Always check your lifestyle, eating, and drinking habits first.

ENEMAS

Enemas are not as bad as they sound. My old-fashioned Italian mother would always insist on an enema when any of her children was sick with a fever. I always thought she was being unreasonable until I realized that what she was doing was cooling down the body from the inside out and eliminating any built-up waste, thus freeing up more energy to be available for healing. I have since carried this practice over to my own two children and have had repeatedly good results. Since my daughters first experienced enemas as very young children, there was less embarrassment and self-consciousness when they got older. It was just accepted as something to be done to encourage recovery.

There are two types of enemas: (1) cleansing, which helps

stimulate the evacuation of the waste in the colon, and (2) retention, which are usually held for approximately fifteen minutes after cleansing to stimulate detoxification and to loosen any encrusted fecal matter that may have built up on the intestinal walls. The cleansing enema is appropriate for occasional constipation. If one is seriously constipated, very often a gentle enema will stimulate evacuation by slightly distending the colon and having the water work as a lubricant around the fecal matter. Usually the stools are hard and dry, so this coaxing brings forth quick relief. A small amount of body-temperature water is slowly placed in the rectum. Far less is needed or tolerated than with a retention enema, as the colon is already filled with waste and cannot hold quite as much. Shortly there will be an urge to evacuate, and you can make the common "run" for relief. If a second enema is needed, it can be repeated immediately after the initial evacuation. Remember this is not something that should be done on a daily or even weekly basis. The amounts of normal water absorption will be thrown off and the bowel will learn to rely on this for elimination rather than normal peristaltic action. But occasional use is okay, providing there is no rectal bleeding. If there is, see a physician immediately and do not take an enema. Another caveat: Be careful not to tear the delicate tissue around the anus, especially if you have hemorrhoids.

CONCLUSION

The tips outlined in this book are intended to act as a guide to a healthier life and to quell the desire to search for a quick fix. Remember that all things worth having are worth working for, including good health. You are worth the extra effort.

BIBLIOGRAPHY

Altomare, D., et al. "Grading the Severity of Chronic Idiopathic Constipation." *Centro Servizi Genius* (January 1996).

Balch, James F., and A. Phyllis. *Prescription for Nutritional Healing,* second edition. New York: Avery, 1997.

Bostick Reed, Patsy. *Nutrition: An Applied Science.* New York: West Publishing, 1980.

Buenos, Hermann. *Uninvited Guests.* Los Angeles: Keats, 1996.

Cavallini, G., et al. "Medical Therapy of Chronic Idiopathic Constipation." *Chirurgia Italiana* 45, no. 1-6, (February-December 1993): 3–28.

Celik, A. F., J. Tomlin, and N. W. Read. "The Effect of Oral Vancomycin on Chronic Idiopathic Constipation." *Alimentary Pharmocological Therapies* 9, no. 1 (February 1995): 63– 68.

Cheskin, L. J., et al. "Mechanisms of Constipation in Older Persons and Effects of Fiber Compared with Placebo." *Journal of American Geriatric Society* 43, no. 6 (June 1995): 666–69.

DiLorenzo, C., et al. "Age-Related Changes in Colon Motility." *Journal of Pediatrics* 127, no. 4 (October 1995): 593–96.

Dincin Buchman, D. *Ancient Healing Secrets.* New York: Random House, 1996.

Duncan, A., et al. "Diagnosis of the Abuse of Magnesium and Stimulant Laxatives." *Annals of Clinical Biochemistry* 28, pt. 6 (November 1991): 568–73.

Gates, Donna, and Linda Schatz. *The Body Ecology Diet.* Atlanta, Georgia: B.E.D. Publications, 1993.

Gibbons, DeLamar. *The Self-Help Way to Treat Colitis and Other I.B.S. Conditions.* Los Angeles: Keats, 1992.

Gwee, K. A., and J. Y. Kang. "Surreptitious Laxative Abuse—An Unusual Cause of Chronic Diarrhoea." *Singapore Medical Journal* 31, no. 6 (December 1990): 596–98.

Hall, G. R., et al. "Managing Constipation Using a Research-Based Protocol." *Medical/Surgical Nursing* 4, no. 1 (February 1995): 8–11, 19–20.

Harar, D., et al. "Correlates of Regular Laxative Use by Frail Elderly Persons." *American Journal of Medicine* 99, no. 5 (1995): 513–18.

Hillemeier, C. "An Overview of the Effects of Dietary Fiber on Gastrointestinal Transit." *Pediatrics* 96, no. 5, pt. 2 (November 1995): 997–99.

Kuwaki, T. *Chinese Herbal Therapy: A Guide to Its Principles and Practices*. Long Beach, Calif.: Ohai Press, 1990.

Lipski, Elizabeth. *Digestive Wellness*. Los Angeles: Keats, 1996.

Mowrey, D. B. *The Scientific Validation of Herbal Medicine*. Los Angeles: Keats, 1986.

Muller, M., et al. "Treatment of Constipation in Pregnant Women. A Multicenter Study in a Gynecological Practice." *Schweizerische Medizinische Wochenschrift* 125, no. 36 (September 9, 1995): 1689–93.

Nyska, A., et al. "Constipation and Megacolon in Rats Related to Treatment with Oxodipine, a Calcium Antagonist." *Toxicologic Pathology* 22, no. 6 (November–December, 1994): 589–94.

Rector-Page, Linda G. *Healthy Healing: An Alternative Healing Reference*. Carmel Valley, Calif.: Healthy Healing Publications, 1992.

Santillo, Humberto. *Natural Healing with Herbs*. Prescott Valley, Ariz.: Hohm Press, 1985.

Shafik, A. "Constipation, Pathogenesis and Management." *Drugs* 45, no. 4 (April 1993): 528–40.

Sieger, C. P., et al. "Anthranoid Laxative Abuse—A Risk for Colorectal Cancer?" *Gut* 34, no. 8 (August 1993): 1099–101.

Vincent, R., et al. "Effect of Bran Particle Size on Gastric Emptying and Small Bowel Transit in Humans: A Scintigraphic Study." *Gut* 37, no. 2 (August 1995): 216–19.

Wu, W. J., et al. "Urolithiasis Related to Laxative Abuse." *Journal Formos Medical Association* 92, no. 11 (November 1993): 1004–6.

www.ingramcontent.com/pod-product-compliance
Ingram Content Group UK Ltd.
Pitfield, Milton Keynes, MK11 3LW, UK
UKHW021502281225
466417UK00025B/50